DOSHA DINING: 300 RECIPES FOR BALANCED WELLNESS

Welcome to "Dosha Dining," a comprehensive culinary journey embracing the principles of Ayurveda. This book offers a delectable array of 300 recipes, thoughtfully curated to balance and harmonize the unique constitutions of Vata, Pitta, and Kapha. Ayurveda, the ancient science of life, recognizes the individual nature of our bodies and minds, emphasizing the significance of harmonizing our doshas—Vata, Pitta, and Kapha—to promote overall well-being.

Each recipe within these pages is meticulously crafted to cater to the distinctive needs of each dosha. Vata individuals, often creative and enthusiastic, benefit from warming and grounding ingredients. Pitta individuals, driven and goal-oriented, thrive on cooling and calming flavors. Kapha individuals, nurturing and steady, find balance in stimulating and light ingredients. These recipes aim to balance the doshas, promoting health, vitality, and balance in mind and body.

Whether you're seeking to balance your dosha or simply enjoy a diverse range of flavors and culinary experiences, "Dosha Dining" invites you on a flavorful odyssey, celebrating the art of cooking tailored to individual constitutions. Explore the pages, engage your senses, and embark on a journey toward holistic well-being through the pleasure of cooking and eating in harmony with your unique self.

TABLE OF CONTENTS

Chapter 1: Pitta-Balancing Recipes

Chapter 2: Vata-Balancing Recipes

Chapter 3: Kapha-Balancing Recipes

Chapter 4: All Doshas-Balancing Recipes

CHAPTER 1: PITTA-BALANCING RECIPES

Pitta dosha is associated with fire, governing digestion and metabolism. The recipes in this section are carefully curated to pacify Pitta, fostering balance and harmony within the body. They feature cooling, soothing, and nourishing ingredients that aid in calming the fiery nature of Pitta dosha.

The chapter delves into a diverse array of 100 recipes specifically tailored to suit individuals with a dominant Pitta dosha. From refreshing beverages to comforting mains and desserts, each recipe is meticulously crafted with ingredients and cooking methods that align with the characteristics of Pitta dosha. The selection includes meals that are light, cooling, and easily digestible, promoting a sense of balance, vitality, and ease within the body.

Detailed instructions accompany each recipe, guiding readers through the preparation process. Emphasis is placed on incorporating cooling herbs, seasonal produce, and mindful cooking techniques to pacify Pitta dosha, fostering not just a delightful dining experience but also overall well-being.

The chapter aims to empower readers to embrace a Pitta-balancing diet and lifestyle, encouraging them to explore the delicious realm of Ayurvedic cooking while harnessing the principles of balance and health.

Pitta dosha-balancing recipes along with a brief on when they might be best enjoyed:

1. **Coconut Chia Seed Pudding:**
    1. Instructions: Mix chia seeds with coconut milk, refrigerate overnight, and serve with fresh fruits.
    2. Time to Eat: Best enjoyed as a cool breakfast.

2. **Cucumber Mint Raita:**
    1. Instructions: Combine diced cucumber with yogurt, chopped mint, cumin, and salt.
    2. Time to Eat: Ideal for lunch, served alongside rice or as a side dish.

3. **Grilled Vegetable Salad:**
    1. Instructions: Grill zucchini, bell peppers, and eggplant; dress with a cooling vinaigrette.
    2. Time to Eat: Perfect for a light dinner option.

4. **Quinoa Stuffed Bell Peppers:**
    1. Instructions: Fill halved bell peppers with a cooked quinoa mix of veggies and herbs.
    2. Time to Eat: Suitable for lunch or a light early dinner.

5. **Spinach Lentil Soup:**
    1. Instructions: Cook lentils and spinach together with cooling spices like coriander and fennel.
    2. Time to Eat: Best as a lunch option.

6. **Mango Lassi:**

    1. Instructions: Blend ripe mangoes with yogurt and a splash of rose water.
    2. Time to Eat: A perfect cooling beverage for mid-morning or afternoon.

7. **Basil Pesto Pasta:**
    1. Instructions: Toss whole-grain pasta with homemade basil pesto, cherry tomatoes, and pine nuts.
    2. Time to Eat: Suitable for lunch or an early dinner.

8. **Cilantro Lime Rice:**
    1. Instructions: Cook rice with lime zest and juice, chopped cilantro, and a touch of ghee.
    2. Time to Eat: Enjoy it as a part of lunch or dinner.

9. **Stir-Fried Tofu with Asparagus:**
    1. Instructions: Stir-fry tofu and asparagus with a hint of sesame oil and ginger.
    2. Time to Eat: Recommended for an early dinner.

10. **Watermelon Feta Salad:**
    1. Instructions: Combine cubed watermelon with feta, mint, and a light vinaigrette.
    2. Time to Eat: Perfect for a refreshing and light dinner option.

11. **Stuffed Bitter Melon (Karela):**
    1. Instructions: Stuff bitter melon with spiced lentil or quinoa mixture, then pan-fry or bake until cooked.
    2. Time to Eat: Best as a part of lunch or dinner.

12. **Cooling Cucumber Soup:**
    1. Instructions: Blend peeled cucumbers with yogurt, dill, and a dash of lemon, chill before

serving.

2. Time to Eat: Ideal for a light lunch or a refreshing mid-afternoon meal.

13. **Tofu Summer Rolls:**

1. Instructions: Wrap tofu, julienned veggies, and fresh herbs in rice paper sheets, served with a tangy peanut dipping sauce.
2. Time to Eat: Perfect as a light dinner or a mid-afternoon snack.

14. **Turmeric Ginger Carrot Soup:**

1. Instructions: Cook carrots with turmeric and ginger, then blend to a smooth consistency.
2. Time to Eat: Suitable for lunch or a light dinner.

15. **Minty Green Pea Hummus:**

1. Instructions: Blend green peas, fresh mint, tahini, and lemon juice for a cooling twist on traditional hummus.
2. Time to Eat: Enjoy as a mid-morning or mid-afternoon snack.

16. **Quinoa Tabbouleh Salad:**

1. Instructions: Toss cooked quinoa with chopped parsley, tomatoes, cucumbers, and a lemony dressing.
2. Time to Eat: Great for a light lunch or an early dinner.

17. **Chickpea Spinach Stir-Fry:**

1. Instructions: Sauté chickpeas and spinach with cooling spices like coriander and a hint of lemon.
2. Time to Eat: Suitable for lunch or a light early dinner.

18. **Sesame Ginger Noodles:**
    1. Instructions: Toss cooked noodles with a sesame-ginger sauce, mixed with shredded veggies.
    2. Time to Eat: Ideal for a light dinner.

19. **Peach Basil Sorbet:**
    1. Instructions: Blend ripe peaches with fresh basil and a touch of honey, then freeze until slushy.
    2. Time to Eat: A delightful dessert for any time of the day.

20. **Chilled Dill Beet Soup:**
    1. Instructions: Blend cooked beets with dill, yogurt, and a hint of garlic, serve chilled.
    2. Time to Eat: Perfect as a cool, refreshing lunch option.

21. **Cauliflower "Fried Rice":**
    1. Instructions: Pulse cauliflower in a food processor, sauté with peas, carrots, and eggs, seasoned lightly with soy sauce and ginger.
    2. Time to Eat: Great for an early dinner.

22. **Cooling Avocado & Cucumber Sushi Rolls:**
    1. Instructions: Create sushi rolls with avocado, cucumber, and quinoa instead of rice, served with a tamari dipping sauce.
    2. Time to Eat: Perfect for lunch or a light dinner.

23. **Minty Watermelon Salad:**
    1. Instructions: Toss cubed watermelon with feta, mint leaves, a drizzle of olive oil, and a pinch of salt.
    2. Time to Eat: Enjoy as a mid-afternoon snack or a refreshing side dish.

24. **Lemon Asparagus Risotto:**
    1. Instructions: Cook risotto with a hint of lemon zest, incorporating asparagus for a cooling effect.
    2. Time to Eat: Ideal for a mid-afternoon meal or an early dinner.

25. **Chickpea Spinach Burgers:**
    1. Instructions: Blend chickpeas, spinach, and cooling spices into patties, then grill or bake until cooked through.
    2. Time to Eat: Perfect for a light dinner.

26. **Green Lentil Salad with Citrus Dressing:**
    1. Instructions: Toss cooked green lentils with mixed greens and a citrusy vinaigrette.
    2. Time to Eat: Great for lunch or a light dinner.

27. **Chilled Melon Soup:**
    1. Instructions: Blend honeydew or cantaloupe with a touch of lime and mint, then chill before serving.
    2. Time to Eat: Ideal for a mid-morning snack or a light dessert.

28. **Coconut Lime Quinoa:**
    1. Instructions: Cook quinoa with coconut milk, lime zest, and a sprinkle of shredded coconut.
    2. Time to Eat: Suitable for lunch or an early dinner.

29. **Parsley Walnut Pesto Pasta:**
    1. Instructions: Toss cooked whole-grain pasta with a parsley-walnut pesto, cherry tomatoes, and a squeeze of lemon.
    2. Time to Eat: Perfect for a light dinner

30. **Apricot Almond Smoothie:**

1. Instructions: Blend apricots, almond milk, a hint of cardamom, and a drizzle of honey until smooth.
2. Time to Eat: Enjoy as a mid-morning or afternoon snack.

31. Mint Cucumber Gazpacho:

1. Instructions: Blend cucumber, mint, bell peppers, and tomatoes, then chill before serving.
2. Time to Eat: Ideal for a light lunch or a mid-afternoon snack.

32. Mung Bean Coconut Curry:

1. Instructions: Cook mung beans with coconut milk, curry spices, and serve over brown rice.
2. Time to Eat: Great for a light dinner.

33. Arugula Peach Salad:

1. Instructions: Toss arugula, peach slices, goat cheese, and a light vinaigrette.
2. Time to Eat: Suitable for lunch or as a side dish.

34. Sweet Potato & Quinoa Stew:

1. Instructions: Combine sweet potatoes, quinoa, carrots, and kale in a vegetable broth, seasoned with cooling spices.
2. Time to Eat: Perfect for a light dinner.

35. Cucumber Tofu Summer Salad:

1. Instructions: Toss sliced cucumbers, marinated tofu, cherry tomatoes, and a light sesame dressing.
2. Time to Eat: Ideal for a light lunch.

36. Zucchini Noodles with Pesto:

1. Instructions: Toss zucchini noodles with a

homemade pesto made from basil, pine nuts, and olive oil.
2. Time to Eat: Suitable for lunch or a light early dinner.

37. Pineapple Mint Smoothie:
1. Instructions: Blend pineapple chunks, mint leaves, yogurt, and a touch of honey until smooth.
2. Time to Eat: Enjoy as a refreshing mid-morning or afternoon snack.

38. Stuffed Bell Peppers with Millet:
1. Instructions: Fill bell peppers with cooked millet, roasted veggies, and herbs, bake until tender.
2. Time to Eat: Perfect for lunch or an early dinner.

39. Apricot Ginger Chutney:
1. Instructions: Cook apricots with ginger, cinnamon, and a hint of honey until softened.
2. Time to Eat: Ideal as a condiment or a mid-afternoon snack.

40. Pomegranate Mint Iced Tea:
1. Instructions: Brew mint tea, chill, and add fresh pomegranate juice, served over ice.
2. Time to Eat: Enjoy as a mid-morning or afternoon beverage.

41. Peach Basil Bruschetta:
3. Instructions: Toast slices of whole-grain bread, top with chopped peaches, basil, a drizzle of balsamic glaze.
4. Time to Eat: Ideal for a mid-morning snack or a light appetizer.

42. Lemon Herb Grilled Tofu:
1. Instructions: Marinate tofu in a mix of lemon juice, herbs, and olive oil, then grill until golden.
2. Time to Eat: Perfect for a light dinner.

44. Minty Green Bean Salad:
1. Instructions: Blanch green beans, toss with chopped mint, almonds, and a light lemon dressing.
2. Time to Eat: Suitable for lunch or a light dinner.

45. Chilled Cantaloupe Soup:
1. Instructions: Blend ripe cantaloupe with a dash of ginger and mint, then chill before serving.
2. Time to Eat: Enjoy as a mid-afternoon snack or a light starter.

46. Carrot Ginger Rice Pilaf:
1. Instructions: Cook rice with grated carrots, ginger, and a pinch of turmeric for a cooling effect.
2. Time to Eat: Ideal for a light lunch or early dinner.

47. Honeydew Cucumber Salsa:
1. Instructions: Combine diced honeydew and cucumber with jalapeño, lime juice, and cilantro.
2. Time to Eat: Suitable as a mid-morning snack or as a side with meals.

48. Millet-Stuffed Portobello Mushrooms:
1. Instructions: Fill portobello mushrooms with cooked millet, spinach, and herbs, then bake until tender.

2. Time to Eat: Great for a light dinner.

49. Cilantro Lime Grilled Corn:

1. Instructions: Grill corn on the cob, then brush with a mix of cilantro, lime, and a touch of butter.
2. Time to Eat: Perfect for a mid-afternoon snack or as a side dish.

50. Watermelon Feta Skewers:

1. Instructions: Thread watermelon cubes and feta on skewers, drizzle with a balsamic glaze.
2. Time to Eat: Enjoy as a light appetizer or a mid-afternoon snack.

51. Apricot Cardamom Compote:

1. Instructions: Simmer apricots with cardamom and a touch of honey until soft.
2. Time to Eat: Ideal as a condiment or a light dessert.

52. Cooling Quinoa Salad:

1. Instructions: Mix cooked quinoa with diced cucumber, fennel, and a lemony dressing.
2. Time to Eat: Ideal for lunch or a light early dinner.

53. Zesty Orange Carrot Soup:

1. Instructions: Blend cooked carrots with orange zest, ginger, and a hint of turmeric, then simmer until warm.
2. Time to Eat: Suitable for lunch or a light dinner.

54. Cucumber Dill Yogurt Dip:

1. Instructions: Combine diced cucumber and fresh dill with yogurt, serve with veggie sticks.

    2. Time to Eat: Perfect as a mid-morning or mid-afternoon snack.

55. Cherry Almond Couscous Salad:

    1. Instructions: Toss cooked couscous with cherries, almonds, and a touch of honey.

    2. Time to Eat: Suitable for lunch or a light early dinner.

56. Mint Watermelon Granita:

    1. Instructions: Blend watermelon with mint, freeze, then scrape with a fork to create a granita.

    2. Time to Eat: Enjoy as a light dessert or a mid-afternoon refresher.

57. Asparagus Basil Risotto:

    1. Instructions: Cook risotto with asparagus and fresh basil, seasoned lightly with lemon.

    2. Time to Eat: Great for a light dinner.

58. Strawberry Arugula Salad:

    1. Instructions: Toss arugula with sliced strawberries, goat cheese, and a balsamic vinaigrette.

    2. Time to Eat: Ideal for lunch or as a side dish.

59. Turmeric Honey Roasted Carrots:

    1. Instructions: Roast carrots with a drizzle of honey and a sprinkle of turmeric.

    2. Time to Eat: Suitable for an early dinner.

60. Mango Basil Salsa:

    1. Instructions: Combine diced mango with fresh basil, jalapeño, lime juice, and red onion.

    2. Time to Eat: Perfect as a light appetizer or a mid-afternoon snack.

61. Papaya Lime Smoothie:

1. Instructions: Blend papaya, lime juice, a hint of coconut milk, and a touch of honey.
2. Time to Eat: Enjoy as a mid-morning or afternoon refresher.

62. Mango Coconut Rice:

1. Instructions: Cook rice in coconut milk, add diced mango and a sprinkle of cardamom.
2. Time to Eat: Great for lunch or an early dinner.

63. Lemon Mint Lentil Salad:

1. Instructions: Toss cooked lentils with fresh mint, lemon zest, and a drizzle of olive oil.
2. Time to Eat: Suitable for lunch or a light dinner.

64. Cauliflower Tabouleh:

1. Instructions: Pulse cauliflower into rice-like grains, mix with chopped parsley, tomatoes, and lemon juice.
2. Time to Eat: Ideal for a light lunch or a mid-afternoon snack.

65. Pomegranate Pistachio Quinoa:

1. Instructions: Mix cooked quinoa with pomegranate arils, chopped pistachios, and a squeeze of lime.
2. Time to Eat: Suitable for lunch or an early dinner.

66. Apricot Basil Chickpea Salad:

1. Instructions: Combine chickpeas with diced apricots, fresh basil, and a light vinaigrette.
2. Time to Eat: Perfect for lunch or a light dinner.

67. Coconut Lime Tofu Stir-Fry:

1. Instructions: Sauté tofu with bell peppers, snow peas, in a coconut-lime sauce.

2. Time to Eat: Great for an early dinner.

68. Arugula Pineapple Salad:

1. Instructions: Toss arugula with pineapple chunks, feta cheese, and a balsamic vinaigrette.
2. Time to Eat: Suitable for lunch or as a refreshing side.

69. Chilled Beetroot Soup:

1. Instructions: Blend cooked beets with Greek yogurt, dill, and a hint of garlic, then chill.
2. Time to Eat: Ideal for a light lunch or a mid-afternoon snack.

70. Cumin Carrot Millet Pilaf:

1. Instructions: Cook millet with cumin-infused carrots, sprinkle with fresh cilantro.
2. Time to Eat: Suitable for lunch or an early dinner.

71. Peach Mint Iced Tea:

1. Instructions: Brew mint tea, blend with fresh peach juice, and serve over ice.
2. Time to Eat: Enjoy as a mid-morning or afternoon beverage.

72. Coconut Lime Tofu Stir-Fry:

1. Instructions: Sauté tofu with bell peppers, snow peas, in a coconut-lime sauce.
2. Time to Eat: Great for an early dinner.

73. Arugula Pineapple Salad:

1. Instructions: Toss arugula with pineapple chunks, feta cheese, and a balsamic vinaigrette.
2. Time to Eat: Suitable for lunch or as a refreshing side.

74. **Chilled Beetroot Soup:**

1. Instructions: Blend cooked beets with Greek yogurt, dill, and a hint of garlic, then chill.
2. Time to Eat: Ideal for a light lunch or a mid-afternoon snack.

75. **Cumin Carrot Millet Pilaf:**

1. Instructions: Cook millet with cumin-infused carrots, sprinkle with fresh cilantro.
2. Time to Eat: Suitable for lunch or an early dinner.

76. **Peach Mint Iced Tea:**

1. Instructions: Brew mint tea, blend with fresh peach juice, and serve over ice.
2. Time to Eat: Enjoy as a mid-morning or afternoon beverage.

77. **Pistachio Mint Quinoa Salad:**

1. Instructions: Mix cooked quinoa with chopped pistachios, fresh mint, and a lemon vinaigrette.
2. Time to Eat: Ideal for lunch or a light early dinner.

78. **Chilled Carrot Ginger Soup:**

1. Instructions: Blend cooked carrots with fresh ginger, yogurt, and a dash of honey, then chill.
2. Time to Eat: Great for a refreshing mid-afternoon snack or a light lunch.

79. **Tomato Basil Bruschetta:**

1. Instructions: Top whole-grain bread with diced tomatoes, fresh basil, and a sprinkle of balsamic vinegar.
2. Time to Eat: Perfect for a light appetizer or a mid-afternoon snack.

80. **Mango Avocado Salsa:**
    1. Instructions: Combine diced mango, avocado, red onion, cilantro, and lime juice.
    2. Time to Eat: Suitable as a light appetizer or a mid-afternoon snack.

81. **Coconut Lime Asparagus:**
    1. Instructions: Sauté asparagus with a coconut-lime glaze and shredded coconut.
    2. Time to Eat: Ideal for a light dinner.

82. **Chickpea Cilantro Cauliflower Rice:**
    1. Instructions: Pulse cauliflower into rice, sauté with chickpeas, fresh cilantro, and cumin.
    2. Time to Eat: Suitable for lunch or an early dinner.

83. **Apricot Almond Couscous:**
    1. Instructions: Cook couscous with dried apricots, toasted almonds, and a hint of almond oil.
    2. Time to Eat: Perfect for a light lunch or a mid-afternoon snack.

84. **Arugula Pomegranate Salad:**
    1. Instructions: Toss arugula with pomegranate arils, goat cheese, and a citrusy vinaigrette.
    2. Time to Eat: Suitable for lunch or a light dinner.

85. **Peach Basil Quinoa Bowl:**
    1. Instructions: Combine cooked quinoa with sliced peaches, fresh basil, and a touch of honey.
    2. Time to Eat: Ideal for lunch or an early dinner.

86. **Chilled Melon Mint Soup:**
    1. Instructions: Blend honeydew melon with

mint leaves, a splash of lime, and chill before serving.

2. Time to Eat: Enjoy as a refreshing mid-afternoon snack or a light dessert.

87. Pineapple Coconut Quinoa:

1. Instructions: Cook quinoa in coconut milk, mix in pineapple chunks, and a sprinkle of shredded coconut.
2. Time to Eat: Ideal for lunch or an early dinner.

88. Chilled Tomato Cucumber Gazpacho:

1. Instructions: Blend tomatoes, cucumbers, bell peppers, and onions, chill before serving.
2. Time to Eat: Great for a refreshing mid-afternoon snack or a light lunch.

89. Minty Pea Hummus:

1. Instructions: Blend peas, fresh mint, tahini, and lemon juice for a cool twist on hummus.
2. Time to Eat: Suitable for a mid-morning or mid-afternoon snack.

90. Lemon Turmeric Roasted Cauliflower:

1. Instructions: Roast cauliflower with a mix of turmeric, lemon zest, and olive oil.
2. Time to Eat: Perfect for a light dinner.

91. Cilantro Lime Zucchini Noodles:

1. Instructions: Toss zucchini noodles with a cilantro-lime dressing and cherry tomatoes.
2. Time to Eat: Ideal for lunch or an early dinner.

92. Apricot Spinach Salad:

1. Instructions: Toss baby spinach with diced apricots, almonds, and a light vinaigrette.
2. Time to Eat: Suitable for lunch or a light dinner.

93. Pomegranate Mint Quinoa Salad:

1. Instructions: Combine cooked quinoa with pomegranate seeds, fresh mint, and a citrusy dressing.
2. Time to Eat: Perfect for a light lunch or an early dinner.

94. Chilled Cantaloupe Basil Soup:

1. Instructions: Blend cantaloupe with fresh basil, chill thoroughly before serving.
2. Time to Eat: Ideal for a refreshing mid-afternoon snack or a light lunch.

95. Mango Turmeric Tofu Stir-Fry:

1. Instructions: Stir-fry tofu with mango cubes, turmeric, and a splash of tamari.
2. Time to Eat: Suitable for an early dinner.

96. Watermelon Feta Mint Salad:

1. Instructions: Combine cubed watermelon, feta, fresh mint, and a drizzle of balsamic glaze.
2. Time to Eat: Great for a light lunch or a mid-afternoon snack.

97. Lemon Basil Grilled Chicken:

1. Instructions: Marinate chicken in a mix of lemon, fresh basil, and grill until fully cooked.
2. Time to Eat: Ideal for an early dinner.

98. Peach Avocado Salsa:

1. Instructions: Combine diced peaches, avocados, red onions, cilantro, and lime juice.
2. Time to Eat: Suitable as a light appetizer or a mid-afternoon snack.

99. Arugula Pine Nut Pasta:

1. Instructions: Toss arugula and pine nuts with

whole-grain pasta and a lemony dressing.
2. Time to Eat: Perfect for a light dinner.

100. **Turmeric Mango Smoothie:**
1. Instructions: Blend mango chunks with a hint of turmeric and coconut milk.
2. Time to Eat: Great for a mid-morning or afternoon snack.

101. **Chilled Beetroot Walnut Salad:**
1. Instructions: Toss cooked beets with walnuts, a touch of olive oil, and fresh dill.
2. Time to Eat: Ideal for lunch or a light early dinner.

These recipes are crafted to balance Pitta dosha; adjust the timing to suit personal eating habits and comfort.

CHAPTER 2: VATA-BALANCING RECIPES

Vata-Balancing Recipes, the focus is on culinary creations specifically designed to balance and soothe Vata dosha. Vata dosha is characterized by qualities of dryness, coldness, lightness, and mobility. It's associated with the air and ether elements. When out of balance, Vata can lead to anxiety, dry skin, and digestive issues.

This section presents a range of recipes tailored to pacify and ground Vata, focusing on ingredients and cooking methods that counter Vata's inherent qualities.

Each recipe is carefully curated with ingredients and cooking methods that align with Vata's needs, such as using warming spices, cooked foods, and hydrating elements to counterbalance Vata's dryness. Additionally, it may include a variety of textures, aromas, and flavors to stimulate and ground the Vata individual.

The chapter not only provides recipes but also educates the reader on the reasoning behind the ingredients and methods used, helping individuals understand how food can be used as a tool to harmonize their doshas for overall well-being.

Vata-balancing recipes involves a diverse selection of dishes and flavors. Here's a selection of recipes specifically curated to balance Vata dosha:

1. **Spiced Oatmeal with Almonds and Dates:**
    1. Instructions: Cook oats with warming spices (cinnamon, cardamom), top with chopped almonds, dates, and a drizzle of ghee or coconut oil.
    2. Time to Eat: Ideal for breakfast to provide warmth and nourishment.

2. **Butternut Squash and Ginger Soup:**
    1. Instructions: Simmer butternut squash with fresh ginger, turmeric, and a hint of coconut milk, then blend until smooth.
    2. Time to Eat: Suitable for lunch, offering grounding warmth.

3. **Cumin-Spiced Lentil Stew:**
    1. Instructions: Cook lentils with cumin, coriander, and a touch of tomato, serve with a side of brown rice.
    2. Time to Eat: Perfect for a grounding dinner.

4. **Sweet Potato and Chickpea Curry:**
    1. Instructions: Simmer sweet potatoes and chickpeas in a blend of warming spices, serve with quinoa or naan bread.
    2. Time to Eat: Great for a nourishing dinner.

5. **Cinnamon Apple Pancakes:**
    1. Instructions: Make pancakes with spelt flour, cinnamon, and chopped apples, serve with a dollop of warm honey or fruit compote.

2. Time to Eat: Ideal for a cozy breakfast.

6. **Roasted Root Vegetable Medley:**
    1. Instructions: Roast a mix of root veggies (carrots, parsnips, beets) with rosemary, olive oil, and a sprinkle of sea salt.
    2. Time to Eat: Suitable for lunch, offering comforting sustenance.

7. **Turmeric Milk with Honey:**
    1. Instructions: Warm milk with turmeric, a touch of honey, and a sprinkle of nutmeg.
    2. Time to Eat: Great for a calming pre-bedtime drink.

8. **Miso-Glazed Eggplant with Quinoa:**
    1. Instructions: Marinate eggplant in miso, roast, and serve with cooked quinoa and a sprinkle of sesame seeds.
    2. Time to Eat: Suitable for a grounding dinner.

9. **Pumpkin and Walnut Loaf:**
    1. Instructions: Bake a loaf with pumpkin puree, chopped walnuts, and a hint of nutmeg.
    2. Time to Eat: Ideal for a comforting snack.

10. **Warm Quinoa Salad with Roasted Vegetables:**
    1. Instructions: Toss cooked quinoa with roasted veggies (zucchini, bell peppers) and a light lemon-tahini dressing.
    2. Time to Eat: Great for a nourishing lunch.

11. **Ghee-Roasted Brussels Sprouts with Pomegranate Seeds:**
    1. Instructions: Roast brussels sprouts in ghee, top with pomegranate seeds and a dash of balsamic glaze.
    2. Time to Eat: Suitable for a dinner side dish.

12. **Date and Nut Energy Balls:**
    1. Instructions: Blend dates, nuts, and a touch of coconut oil, roll into balls and coat with shredded coconut.
    2. Time to Eat: Ideal for a quick, grounding snack.

13. **Cardamom-Spiced Rice Pudding:**
    1. Instructions: Cook rice with cardamom, add milk, and a hint of coconut sugar or jaggery.
    2. Time to Eat: Great as a comforting dessert or breakfast option.

14. **Millet and Vegetable Stuffed Peppers:**
    1. Instructions: Stuff bell peppers with cooked millet, sautéed veggies, and a sprinkle of fresh herbs.
    2. Time to Eat: Suitable for a filling dinner.

15. **Cumin Carrot Soup with Coconut Cream:**
    1. Instructions: Simmer carrots with cumin, blend, and top with a swirl of coconut cream.
    2. Time to Eat: Ideal for lunch, offering warmth and nourishment.

16. **Tahini Cauliflower Steaks:**
    1. Instructions: Roast thick cauliflower slices drizzled with tahini, top with toasted sesame seeds.
    2. Time to Eat: Suitable for a grounding dinner.

17. **Almond Butter Banana Smoothie:**
    1. Instructions: Blend almond butter, bananas, dates, and almond milk for a creamy treat.
    2. Time to Eat: Great for a mid-morning or mid-afternoon snack.

18. **Veggie Noodle Stir-Fry with Ginger Sauce:**

1. Instructions: Stir-fry spiralized veggies with a ginger-infused sauce, serve over brown rice.
2. Time to Eat: Ideal for a nourishing dinner.

19. Fig and Walnut Compote with Yogurt:

1. Instructions: Simmer figs and walnuts in a saucepan, serve over yogurt with a sprinkle of cinnamon.
2. Time to Eat: Suitable for a comforting dessert or breakfast.

20. Chai-Spiced Chia Pudding:

1. Instructions: Soak chia seeds in chai spices and almond milk, top with chopped nuts and dried fruits.
2. Time to Eat: Great for a filling breakfast or a comforting dessert option.

21. Turmeric Ginger Carrot Soup:

1. Instructions: Simmer carrots with fresh turmeric, ginger, and coconut milk, then blend until creamy.
2. Time to Eat: Ideal for a warming lunch.

22. Quinoa Pancakes with Maple Syrup:

1. Instructions: Make quinoa pancakes with a drizzle of maple syrup and a side of warm fruit compote.
2. Time to Eat: Perfect for a grounding breakfast.

23. Warm Brussels Sprout Salad:

1. Instructions: Sauté shredded Brussels sprouts with toasted pine nuts and a lemon-tahini dressing.
2. Time to Eat: Suitable for a comforting lunch.

24. Millet Porridge with Sliced Apples:

1. Instructions: Cook millet porridge with

cinnamon, top with sliced apples and a sprinkle of almonds.
2. Time to Eat: Great for a nourishing breakfast.

25. Sesame Crusted Baked Tofu:
1. Instructions: Coat tofu with sesame seeds, bake until crispy, serve with steamed greens.
2. Time to Eat: Suitable for a grounding dinner.

26. Pear and Walnut Muffins:
1. Instructions: Bake muffins using whole wheat flour, pears, walnuts, and a touch of nutmeg.
2. Time to Eat: Ideal for a cozy snack.

27. Warm Spinach Artichoke Dip:
1. Instructions: Mix warm spinach, artichoke hearts, and a blend of creamy cheese, serve with pita chips.
2. Time to Eat: Suitable for a comforting appetizer.

28. Ghee-Roasted Cauliflower Hummus:
1. Instructions: Roast cauliflower, blend with ghee and chickpeas, serve with warm pita bread.
2. Time to Eat: Great for a cozy snack.

29. Lentil Stuffed Acorn Squash:
1. Instructions: Roast acorn squash, stuff with lentils, cranberries, and a hint of nutmeg.
2. Time to Eat: Suitable for a grounding dinner.

30. Cumin Seed Flatbread:
1. Instructions: Make flatbread with whole wheat flour, cumin seeds, and a touch of olive oil.
2. Time to Eat: Ideal for a warming lunch.

31. Chickpea and Roasted Red Pepper Dip:

1. Instructions: Blend chickpeas with roasted red peppers, tahini, and a hint of paprika.
2. Time to Eat: Suitable for a comforting appetizer.

32. **Cashew Apricot Energy Bars:**
    1. Instructions: Blend cashews, apricots, and oats, press into bars, and refrigerate.
    2. Time to Eat: Great for a quick, grounding snack.

33. **Quinoa Salad with Roasted Root Veggies:**
    1. Instructions: Toss cooked quinoa with roasted root vegetables, a lemon-olive oil dressing, and fresh herbs.
    2. Time to Eat: Ideal for a filling lunch.

34. **Warm Baked Apples with Cinnamon:**
    1. Instructions: Bake apples with a sprinkle of cinnamon and a drizzle of honey, serve warm.
    2. Time to Eat: Suitable for a comforting dessert.

35. **Coconut Curry Pumpkin Seeds:**
    1. Instructions: Roast pumpkin seeds in a coconut curry mix until crispy.
    2. Time to Eat: Great for a cozy snack.

36. **Roasted Eggplant and Tomato Stew:**
    1. Instructions: Roast eggplant and tomatoes, simmer with warming spices for a hearty stew.
    2. Time to Eat: Ideal for a grounding dinner.

37. **Oat Flour Blueberry Waffles:**
    1. Instructions: Make waffles using oat flour, blueberries, and a touch of vanilla extract.
    2. Time to Eat: Suitable for a nurturing breakfast.

38. **Rice and Lentil Stuffed Bell Peppers:**
    1. Instructions: Stuff bell peppers with a mix of rice, lentils, and savory spices, bake until tender.
    2. Time to Eat: Great for a filling dinner.

39. **Warm Ginger Chai Tea:**
    1. Instructions: Brew chai tea with fresh ginger, cardamom, and a touch of honey.
    2. Time to Eat: Suitable for a calming afternoon drink.

40. **Warm Apple Cinnamon Rice Pudding:**
    1. Instructions: Cook rice with apples, cinnamon, and a hint of maple syrup for a comforting dessert or breakfast.
    2. Time to Eat: Suitable for a calming afternoon drink.

41. **Cinnamon Almond Breakfast Bars:**
    1. Instructions: Mix rolled oats, almonds, cinnamon, and honey, press into bars, and bake.
    2. Time to Eat: Ideal for a grounding breakfast.

42. **Baked Acorn Squash with Cumin Butter:**
    1. Instructions: Roast acorn squash, top with a cumin-infused butter.
    2. Time to Eat: Suitable for a comforting dinner.

43. **Coconut Cardamom Rice Pudding:**
    1. Instructions: Cook rice with coconut milk, cardamom, and a touch of coconut sugar.
    2. Time to Eat: Great as a comforting dessert.

44. **Veggie Lentil Soup with Turmeric:**
    1. Instructions: Prepare a hearty soup with lentils, veggies, and a sprinkle of turmeric.

2. Time to Eat: Ideal for a warming lunch.

45. Fig and Walnut Quinoa Porridge:

1. Instructions: Cook quinoa with figs, walnuts, and a hint of nutmeg.
2. Time to Eat: Suitable for a grounding breakfast.

46. Roasted Carrot and Orange Salad:

1. Instructions: Roast carrots, toss with orange segments, and a light vinaigrette.
2. Time to Eat: Great for a midday lunch.

47. Almond Butter and Date Smoothie:

1. Instructions: Blend almond butter, dates, and almond milk until creamy.
2. Time to Eat: Ideal for a grounding mid-morning snack.

48. Mushroom and Asparagus Stir-Fry:

1. Instructions: Sauté mushrooms, asparagus with a hint of ginger and tamari.
2. Time to Eat: Suitable for a grounding dinner.

49. Sesame Ginger Bok Choy:

1. Instructions: Sauté bok choy with sesame oil, fresh ginger, and sesame seeds.
2. Time to Eat: Great for a nourishing dinner.

50. Warm Millet and Date Salad:

1. Instructions: Toss cooked millet with chopped dates, almonds, and a citrusy dressing.
2. Time to Eat: Ideal for a comforting lunch.

51. Tahini and Honey Roasted Carrot Fries:

1. Instructions: Bake carrot sticks with a drizzle of tahini and honey until caramelized.
2. Time to Eat: Suitable for a comforting snack.

52. Coconut Curry Lentil Patties:
1. Instructions: Form lentil patties with coconut curry spices, bake until crispy.
2. Time to Eat: Great for a warming lunch.

53. Chia Seed Pudding with Pomegranate:
1. Instructions: Soak chia seeds in almond milk, top with pomegranate seeds.
2. Time to Eat: Ideal for a grounding breakfast or a light dessert.

54. Lemon Scented Roasted Potatoes:
1. Instructions: Roast potatoes with a drizzle of olive oil, lemon zest, and fresh thyme.
2. Time to Eat: Suitable for a nourishing dinner.

55. Cashew Kale Pesto Pasta:
1. Instructions: Blend cashews, kale, olive oil, and garlic, toss with cooked pasta.
2. Time to Eat: Great for a comforting dinner.

56. Honey Nut Baked Apples:
1. Instructions: Core apples, fill with nuts, honey, and bake until soft.
2. Time to Eat: Ideal for a grounding dessert.

57. Cumin Roasted Cauliflower Soup:
1. Instructions: Roast cauliflower with cumin, blend into a creamy soup.
2. Time to Eat: Suitable for a comforting lunch.

58. Apricot Walnut Couscous Salad:
1. Instructions: Mix cooked couscous with dried apricots, walnuts, and a citrus vinaigrette.
2. Time to Eat: Great for a nourishing lunch.

59. Ginger Spiced Baked Pears:
1. Instructions: Bake pears with a sprinkle of

ginger, cinnamon, and a drizzle of maple syrup.
2. Time to Eat: Ideal for a comforting dessert.

60. Coconut Cardamom Rice Balls:

1. Instructions: Mix cooked rice with coconut milk, cardamom, and roll into small balls.
2. Time to Eat: Suitable for a grounding snack.

61. Caramelized Onion and Mushroom Quiche:

1. Instructions: Bake a quiche with caramelized onions, mushrooms, and a hint of thyme.
2. Time to Eat: Ideal for a warming brunch or dinner.

62. Orange Cardamom Chia Pudding:

1. Instructions: Soak chia seeds in orange juice, cardamom, and almond milk, top with orange zest.
2. Time to Eat: Suitable for a grounding breakfast or dessert.

63. Baked Turmeric Tofu with Miso Glaze:

1. Instructions: Marinate tofu in a miso-turmeric mix, bake until golden, serve with a side of steamed greens.
2. Time to Eat: Great for a grounding dinner.

64. Honey Nut Spiced Granola:

1. Instructions: Mix oats, nuts, honey, and warming spices, bake until golden.
2. Time to Eat: Ideal for a comforting breakfast or snack.

65. Roasted Beet and Citrus Salad:

1. Instructions: Roast beets, toss with citrus segments, mixed greens, and a light vinaigrette.

2. Time to Eat: Suitable for a nourishing lunch.

66. Coconut Date Truffles:

1. Instructions: Blend dates and shredded coconut, roll into small truffles and chill.
2. Time to Eat: Great for a grounding dessert or snack.

67. Warm Pumpkin Sage Risotto:

1. Instructions: Cook risotto with pumpkin puree, sage, and a sprinkle of parmesan.
2. Time to Eat: Ideal for a cozy dinner.

68. Cashew Rosemary Roasted Potatoes:

1. Instructions: Roast potatoes with a coating of cashews, rosemary, and olive oil.
2. Time to Eat: Suitable for a comforting side dish.

69. Sesame Ginger Green Beans:

1. Instructions: Sauté green beans with sesame oil, fresh ginger, and sesame seeds.
2. Time to Eat: Great for a grounding side dish.

70. Maple Cinnamon Baked Bananas:

1. Instructions: Bake bananas with a drizzle of maple syrup, cinnamon, and a sprinkle of nuts.
2. Time to Eat: Ideal for a comforting dessert or breakfast.

71. Lentil and Vegetable Pot Pie:

1. Instructions: Make a pie with lentils, mixed veggies, and a flaky pastry top.
2. Time to Eat: Suitable for a grounding dinner.

72. Honey Cardamom Yogurt Parfait:

1. Instructions: Layer yogurt with honey, cardamom, and a topping of nuts and fruits.

2. Time to Eat: Great for a grounding breakfast or dessert.

73. **Savory Baked Acorn Squash:**
    1. Instructions: Bake acorn squash filled with a mix of rice, vegetables, and savory spices.
    2. Time to Eat: Ideal for a warming dinner.

74. **Apple Walnut Quinoa Bowl:**
    1. Instructions: Mix cooked quinoa with chopped apples, walnuts, and a touch of honey.
    2. Time to Eat: Suitable for a comforting lunch.

75. **Lemon Almond Baked Fish:**
    1. Instructions: Bake fish fillets with a lemon-almond crust until golden.
    2. Time to Eat: Great for a nourishing dinner.

76. **Cumin Roasted Carrot and Parsnip Soup:**
    1. Instructions: Roast carrots and parsnips with cumin, blend into a creamy soup.
    2. Time to Eat: Ideal for a comforting lunch.

77. **Chickpea Spinach Curry with Turmeric:**
    1. Instructions: Prepare a curry with chickpeas, spinach, and a dash of turmeric.
    2. Time to Eat: Suitable for a grounding dinner.

78. **Spiced Date and Nut Butter Toast:**
    1. Instructions: Spread nut butter on toast, top with sliced dates and a sprinkle of warming spices.
    2. Time to Eat: Great for a grounding breakfast or snack.

79. **Cinnamon Raisin Sweet Potato Mash:**
    1. Instructions: Mash sweet potatoes with a hint of cinnamon and raisins.

2. Time to Eat: Ideal for a comforting side dish.

80. **Parsley Cashew Pesto Pasta:**
    1. Instructions: Blend parsley, cashews, and olive oil for a fragrant pasta sauce.
    2. Time to Eat: Suitable for a nurturing dinner.

81. **Turmeric Almond Milk Smoothie:**
    1. Instructions: Blend almond milk with turmeric, a banana, and a hint of honey.
    2. Time to Eat: Ideal for a grounding breakfast or mid-morning snack.

82. **Miso-Glazed Roasted Eggplant:**
    1. Instructions: Roast eggplant brushed with a miso glaze until tender.
    2. Time to Eat: Suitable for a comforting dinner.

83. **Cardamom Spiced Chia Pudding:**
    1. Instructions: Soak chia seeds in cardamom-infused almond milk, top with fresh berries.
    2. Time to Eat: Great for a grounding breakfast or a light dessert.

84. **Warm Lentil and Vegetable Soup:**
    1. Instructions: Prepare a hearty soup with lentils, veggies, and warming spices.
    2. Time to Eat: Ideal for a nurturing lunch.

85. **Roasted Root Vegetables with Thyme:**
    1. Instructions: Roast a medley of root veggies with olive oil, garlic, and thyme.
    2. Time to Eat: Suitable for a comforting dinner.

86. **Warm Quinoa and Fig Porridge:**
    1. Instructions: Cook quinoa with figs, a touch of maple syrup, and chopped nuts.
    2. Time to Eat: Great for a grounding breakfast.

87. **Sesame Ginger Baked Tofu:**
    1. Instructions: Marinate tofu in a sesame ginger sauce and bake until crispy.
    2. Time to Eat: Suitable for a warming dinner.

88. **Rosemary Honey Roasted Carrots:**
    1. Instructions: Roast carrots with rosemary, a drizzle of honey, and a hint of sea salt.
    2. Time to Eat: Ideal for a comforting side dish.

89. **Chickpea Flour Pancakes with Berries:**
    1. Instructions: Make chickpea flour pancakes and top with fresh berries.
    2. Time to Eat: Suitable for a grounding breakfast.

90. **Spinach Walnut Pesto Pasta:**
    1. Instructions: Blend spinach, walnuts, garlic, and olive oil for a nourishing pasta sauce.
    2. Time to Eat: Great for a nurturing dinner.

91. **Lemon Ginger Roasted Broccoli:**
    1. Instructions: Roast broccoli with a lemon-ginger glaze until slightly crispy.
    2. Time to Eat: Ideal for a comforting side dish.

92. **Coconut Cardamom Stuffed Dates:**
    1. Instructions: Stuff dates with a mix of shredded coconut and cardamom, bake until warm.
    2. Time to Eat: Suitable for a grounding dessert or snack.

93. **Cumin Spiced Lentil Patties:**
    1. Instructions: Form lentil patties seasoned with cumin, bake until golden.
    2. Time to Eat: Great for a grounding dinner.

94. **Chai-Spiced Almond Flour Muffins:**

1. Instructions: Bake muffins using almond flour and chai-inspired spices.
2. Time to Eat: Ideal for a comforting snack or breakfast.

95. **Ginger Lemongrass Green Tea:**
     1. Instructions: Brew green tea with fresh ginger and lemongrass for a calming beverage.
     2. Time to Drink: Suitable for a grounding afternoon drink.

96. **Curried Sweet Potato Hash:**
     1. Instructions: Sauté sweet potatoes with a dash of curry powder and herbs.
     2. Time to Eat: Great for a comforting breakfast.

97. **Honey Thyme Roasted Butternut Squash:**
     1. Instructions: Roast butternut squash with a honey-thyme glaze until tender.
     2. Time to Eat: Ideal for a nurturing side dish.

98. **Millet and Date Stuffed Bell Peppers:**
     1. Instructions: Stuff bell peppers with cooked millet, dates, and spices, bake until soft.
     2. Time to Eat: Suitable for a grounding dinner.

99. **Cinnamon Raisin Baked Oatmeal:**
     1. Instructions: Bake an oatmeal dish with cinnamon, raisins, and a touch of maple syrup.
     2. Time to Eat: Great for a comforting breakfast.

100. **Coconut Curry Cauliflower Rice:**
     1. Instructions: Sauté cauliflower rice in a coconut curry sauce with added veggies.
     2. Time to Eat: Suitable for a grounding dinner.

These Vata-balancing recipes encompass a range of meals

and snacks designed to offer grounding, nourishment, and warmth, catering specifically to Vata dosha needs.

Adjust the serving sizes and ingredients based on personal preferences and dietary requirements.

CHAPTER 3: KAPHA-BALANCING RECIPES

et's venture into the realm of Kapha-balancing recipes, designed to invigorate and harmonize the body and mind in accordance with Ayurvedic principles. Kapha, characterized by earthy and watery elements, benefits from meals that embody lightness, warmth, and stimulating flavors. These recipes are crafted to awaken the senses, counterbalance lethargy, and nurture the body, offering a diverse array of tastes and textures to revitalize and balance this dosha. From aromatic spices to vibrant produce, each recipe is a symphony of nourishment and equilibrium, meticulously tailored to cater to the needs of Kapha dosha.

1. **Spicy Lentil Soup:**
   1. Instructions: Prepare a lentil soup with cumin, coriander, and a touch of chili for warmth.
   2. Time to Eat: Ideal for a grounding lunch.

2. **Ginger Lemon Tea:**
   1. Instructions: Brew tea with fresh ginger and a hint of lemon for a refreshing beverage.
   2. Time to Drink: Suitable for a midday pick-me-up.

3. **Roasted Vegetable Quinoa Salad:**

1. Instructions: Toss roasted veggies with quinoa and a tangy vinaigrette.
2. Time to Eat: Great for a nourishing lunch.

4. **Turmeric Cauliflower Steaks:**
   1. Instructions: Roast cauliflower steaks seasoned with turmeric and served with a tangy sauce.
   2. Time to Eat: Ideal for a grounding dinner.

5. **Warm Pear Porridge:**
   1. Instructions: Cook oats with diced pears, cinnamon, and a drizzle of honey.
   2. Time to Eat: Suitable for a comforting breakfast.

6. **Spiced Chickpea Stew:**
   1. Instructions: Prepare a chickpea stew with a mix of warming spices like cinnamon and cloves.
   2. Time to Eat: Great for a filling dinner.

7. **Lemon Thyme Roasted Carrots:**
   1. Instructions: Roast carrots with a lemon-thyme glaze for a zesty side dish.
   2. Time to Eat: Ideal for a comforting side.

8. **Sesame Ginger Tofu Stir-Fry:**
   1. Instructions: Sauté tofu with a sesame-ginger sauce and colorful veggies.
   2. Time to Eat: Suitable for a grounding dinner.

9. **Citrus Beet Salad with Arugula:**
   1. Instructions: Toss roasted beets with fresh citrus segments and peppery arugula.
   2. Time to Eat: Great for a refreshing lunch.

10. **Warm Berry Compote with Almonds:**
    1. Instructions: Simmer berries with a touch of honey, serve warm with toasted almonds.

2. Time to Eat: Ideal for a comforting dessert.

11. Spicy Sweet Potato Wedges:

1. Instructions: Roast sweet potatoes with a spicy seasoning for a warming side.
2. Time to Eat: Suitable for a grounding dinner.

12. Ginger Carrot Muffins:

1. Instructions: Bake muffins with shredded carrots, ginger, and a hint of nutmeg.
2. Time to Eat: Great for a nourishing breakfast or snack.

13. Cumin-Spiced Lentil Salad:

1. Instructions: Toss cooked lentils with cumin, lemon juice, and fresh herbs.
2. Time to Eat: Ideal for a nourishing lunch.

14. Turmeric Cauliflower Soup:

1. Instructions: Blend roasted cauliflower with turmeric for a velvety soup.
2. Time to Eat: Suitable for a comforting dinner.

15. Minty Green Pea Mash:

1. Instructions: Mash green peas with mint and a touch of olive oil for a refreshing side.
2. Time to Eat: Great for a grounding dinner.

16. Warm Date Walnut Porridge:

1. Instructions: Cook oatmeal with chopped dates, walnuts, and a sprinkle of cinnamon.
2. Time to Eat: Ideal for a comforting breakfast.

17. Cinnamon Baked Apple Chips:

1. Instructions: Bake apple slices with a dusting of cinnamon for a wholesome snack.
2. Time to Eat: Suitable for a grounding snack.

18. Lemon Ginger Zucchini Noodles:

1. Instructions: Sauté zucchini noodles with a zesty lemon-ginger dressing.
2. Time to Eat: Great for a refreshing lunch.

19. Coriander Spiced Tomato Soup:

1. Instructions: Prepare a tomato soup with coriander and a hint of paprika.
2. Time to Eat: Ideal for a warming lunch.

20. Spiced Orange Lentil Dip:

1. Instructions: Blend cooked lentils with orange zest, spices, and serve as a dip.
2. Time to Eat: Suitable for a grounding appetizer.

21. Baked Spiced Pears:

1. Instructions: Bake pears with a sprinkle of cinnamon and a touch of honey.
2. Time to Eat: Ideal for a comforting dessert.

22. Saffron Cardamom Rice Pudding:

1. Instructions: Cook rice with saffron, cardamom, and a hint of sweetness.
2. Time to Eat: Suitable for a grounding dessert.

23. Roasted Brussels Sprouts with Mustard Seeds:

1. Instructions: Roast Brussels sprouts with mustard seeds and a squeeze of lemon.
2. Time to Eat: Great for a comforting side dish.

24. Warm Ginger Pear Smoothie:

1. Instructions: Blend pears, fresh ginger, and almond milk until smooth.
2. Time to Eat: Ideal for a grounding breakfast or snack.

25. Turmeric Zucchini Fritters:

1. Instructions: Shred zucchini, mix with turmeric and herbs, fry into fritters.

2. Time to Eat: Suitable for a warming lunch.

26. Citrus Mint Quinoa Salad:

1. Instructions: Toss quinoa with citrus segments, mint, and a light vinaigrette.
2. Time to Eat: Great for a refreshing lunch.

27. Lemon Thyme Baked Chicken:

1. Instructions: Bake chicken with a lemon-thyme marinade until tender.
2. Time to Eat: Ideal for a comforting dinner.

28. Spicy Broccoli Walnut Stir-Fry:

1. Instructions: Sauté broccoli and walnuts with a spicy sauce.
2. Time to Eat: Suitable for a grounding dinner.

29. Ginger Beetroot Detox Juice:

1. Instructions: Juice beets with ginger for a cleansing beverage.
2. Time to Drink: Great for a revitalizing morning drink.

30. Carrot Cumin Soup:

1. Instructions: Cook carrots with cumin, garlic, and blend into a hearty soup.
2. Time to Eat: Ideal for a comforting lunch.

31. Spiced Chickpea Patties:

1. Instructions: Form chickpea patties seasoned with warming spices, bake until crisp.
2. Time to Eat: Suitable for a grounding dinner.

32. Warm Berry Compote with Chia Seeds:

1. Instructions: Simmer berries with chia seeds and a hint of honey, serve warm.
2. Time to Eat: Great for a comforting dessert.

33. Rosemary Citrus Roasted Potatoes:

1. Instructions: Roast potatoes with rosemary, orange zest, and a drizzle of olive oil.
2. Time to Eat: Ideal for a grounding side dish.

34. Warm Walnut Date Scones:

1. Instructions: Bake scones with chopped walnuts, dates, and a touch of cinnamon.
2. Time to Eat: Suitable for a nurturing breakfast.

35. Turmeric Spiced Lentil Curry:

1. Instructions: Prepare a lentil curry with turmeric and a blend of aromatic spices.
2. Time to Eat: Great for a comforting dinner.

36. Citrus Dressed Spinach Salad:

1. Instructions: Toss spinach with a citrusy vinaigrette and toasted almonds.
2. Time to Eat: Ideal for a refreshing lunch.

37. Ginger Papaya Smoothie:

1. Instructions: Blend papaya, fresh ginger, and yogurt for a digestive drink.
2. Time to Drink: Suitable for a grounding morning drink.

38. Cinnamon Baked Sweet Potatoes:

1. Instructions: Bake sweet potatoes with a sprinkle of cinnamon until caramelized.
2. Time to Eat: Great for a comforting side dish.

39. Saffron Cardamom Infused Milk:

1. Instructions: Simmer milk with saffron, cardamom, and a touch of honey.
2. Time to Drink: Ideal for a comforting bedtime drink.

40. Lemon Turmeric Roasted Cauliflower:

1. Instructions: Roast cauliflower with a lemon-

turmeric glaze for a zesty side.
2. Time to Eat: Suitable for a grounding dinner.

41. Warm Cinnamon Raisin Millet Porridge:
1. Instructions: Cook millet with cinnamon, raisins, and a dash of nutmeg.
2. Time to Eat: Ideal for a comforting breakfast.

42. Ginger Lemon Baked Cod:
1. Instructions: Bake cod fillets with a marinade of ginger, lemon, and dill.
2. Time to Eat: Suitable for a grounding dinner.

43. Turmeric Carrot Ginger Soup:
1. Instructions: Blend carrots with ginger and turmeric into a comforting soup.
2. Time to Eat: Great for a nurturing lunch.

44. Spicy Black Bean Tacos:
1. Instructions: Prepare tacos with spiced black beans, fresh salsa, and avocado.
2. Time to Eat: Ideal for a grounding dinner.

45. Rosemary Orange Quinoa Salad:
1. Instructions: Mix cooked quinoa with rosemary, orange segments, and a light dressing.
2. Time to Eat: Suitable for a refreshing lunch.

46. Warm Date Nut Porridge:
1. Instructions: Cook oats with chopped dates, nuts, and a sprinkle of cardamom.
2. Time to Eat: Great for a comforting breakfast.

47. Turmeric Cauliflower Rice Pilaf:
1. Instructions: Sauté cauliflower rice with turmeric, onions, and a mix of spices.
2. Time to Eat: Ideal for a grounding dinner.

48. **Lemon Mint Zucchini Ribbon Salad:**
    1. Instructions: Toss zucchini ribbons with a zesty lemon-mint dressing.
    2. Time to Eat: Suitable for a refreshing lunch.

49. **Spiced Roasted Squash:**
    1. Instructions: Roast squash with a mix of warming spices and a drizzle of olive oil.
    2. Time to Eat: Great for a comforting side dish.

50. **Chai-Spiced Baked Apples:**
    1. Instructions: Bake apples with chai spices until soft and fragrant.
    2. Time to Eat: Ideal for a grounding dessert.

51. **Lentil Kale Tamarind Soup:**
    1. Instructions: Prepare a soup with lentils, kale, and a touch of tangy tamarind.
    2. Time to Eat: Suitable for a nurturing lunch.

52. **Minty Green Pea Hummus:**
    1. Instructions: Blend green peas with mint and spices for a refreshing dip.
    2. Time to Eat: Great for a grounding snack.

53. **Warm Almond Butter Banana Toast:**
    1. Instructions: Toast bread, spread with almond butter, top with banana slices.
    2. Time to Eat: Ideal for a comforting breakfast or snack.

54. **Lemon Turmeric Roasted Asparagus:**
    1. Instructions: Roast asparagus with a lemon-turmeric glaze until tender.
    2. Time to Eat: Suitable for a grounding side dish.

55. **Saffron Date Nut Milk:**
    1. Instructions: Blend dates, nuts, and saffron-

infused milk for a nurturing beverage.

2. Time to Drink: Great for a comforting drink.

56. Ginger Carrot Lentil Salad:

1. Instructions: Toss cooked lentils with ginger, carrots, and a light dressing.
2. Time to Eat: Ideal for a comforting lunch.

57. Cumin Spiced Roasted Cauliflower:

1. Instructions: Roast cauliflower with cumin, coriander, and a hint of chili powder.
2. Time to Eat: Suitable for a grounding dinner.

58. Turmeric Ginger Butternut Squash Soup:

1. Instructions: Blend butternut squash with turmeric, ginger, and a touch of cream.
2. Time to Eat: Great for a comforting lunch.

59. Cardamom Spiced Roasted Nuts:

1. Instructions: Roast mixed nuts with cardamom, sea salt, and a drizzle of honey.
2. Time to Eat: Ideal for a grounding snack.

60. Warm Apple Cinnamon Buckwheat Pancakes:

1. Instructions: Cook buckwheat pancakes with apple slices and a sprinkle of cinnamon.
2. Time to Eat: Suitable for a comforting breakfast.

These Kapha-balancing recipes aim to enliven the palate with flavors that counterbalance Kapha dosha tendencies. Adjust portions and ingredients based on personal preferences and dietary requirements.

CHAPTER 4: ALL DOSHAS-BALANCING RECIPES

1. **Purpose:** This chapter focuses on dishes that cater to the needs of all doshas, promoting balance and harmony within the body. Each recipe is carefully curated to pacify imbalances across all three doshas, nurturing overall well-being.

2. **Recipe Collection:** This section encompasses a diverse array of recipes that bring together ingredients and cooking techniques tailored to create a holistic balance. From energizing breakfast options to satisfying dinners and nourishing snacks, the recipes are carefully crafted to bring equilibrium to the mind, body, and spirit.

3. **Diversity and Harmony:** The recipes in this chapter draw upon various food groups, utilizing a wide array of ingredients that complement and balance each other. Each recipe is designed to offer a blend of tastes – sweet, sour, salty, bitter, pungent, and astringent – ensuring a harmonious blend of flavors.

4. **Adaptable and Versatile:** The recipes are versatile and adaptable to accommodate different dietary needs and preferences. They emphasize a balance of flavors and nutrients, encouraging a holistic approach to

nourishment.

5. **Balancing the Doshas:** Through a meticulous selection of ingredients and mindful preparation, these recipes aim to align the body's natural energies, ensuring that the doshas are in equilibrium. They cater to different seasons and varying individual needs.

6. **Key Highlights:**
   o   Recipes that encompass a variety of tastes and ingredients.
   o   Nourishing and balanced meals suitable for breakfast, lunch, dinner, and snacks.
   o   Emphasis on holistic well-being and maintaining a balanced dosha profile.

7. **Closing Thoughts:** Chapter 4 endeavors to present an amalgamation of flavors and cooking methods that are conducive to balancing the intricate energies of the doshas, offering a guide to fostering overall harmony and well-being.

This chapter amalgamates a diverse selection of recipes that strive to balance and harmonize the individual doshas, catering to the comprehensive well-being of the body and mind.

Here are more recipes that aim to balance all three doshas:

1. **Quinoa Stuffed Bell Peppers:**
   1. Instructions: Fill bell peppers with a mix of quinoa, veggies, and spices, bake until tender.
   2. Time to Eat: Suitable for a grounding dinner.

2. **Baked Eggplant Parmesan:**

1. Instructions: Layer eggplant slices with marinara sauce and cheese, bake until bubbly.
2. Time to Eat: Ideal for a comforting dinner.

3. **Sesame Ginger Green Beans:**
   1. Instructions: Sauté green beans with a sesame-ginger glaze for a flavorful side.
   2. Time to Eat: Suitable for a grounding dinner.

4. **Mango Turmeric Smoothie Bowl:**
   1. Instructions: Blend mango, turmeric, and coconut milk for a vibrant smoothie bowl.
   2. Time to Eat: Ideal for a refreshing breakfast.

5. **Spiced Lentil Stuffed Cabbage Rolls:**
   1. Instructions: Roll cooked lentils in cabbage leaves with a medley of warming spices, bake until tender.
   2. Time to Eat: Suitable for a grounding dinner.

6. **Avocado Cilantro Lime Rice:**
   1. Instructions: Mix cooked rice with mashed avocado, cilantro, and lime juice.
   2. Time to Eat: Ideal for a comforting side dish.

7. **Tofu Veggie Stir-Fry with Brown Rice:**
   1. Instructions: Sauté tofu and assorted vegetables, serve over brown rice with a light soy sauce.
   2. Time to Eat: Suitable for a grounding dinner.

8. **Basil Lemon Chickpea Salad:**
   1. Instructions: Toss chickpeas with fresh basil, lemon zest, and olive oil for a refreshing salad.
   2. Time to Eat: Ideal for a nurturing lunch.

9. **Turmeric Cauliflower Quinoa Bowl:**
   1. Instructions: Roast turmeric cauliflower, serve over quinoa with a sprinkle of herbs.

2. Time to Eat: Suitable for a grounding dinner.

10. Cumin Spiced Sweet Potato Fries:
1. Instructions: Bake sweet potato fries seasoned with cumin and a hint of paprika.
2. Time to Eat: Ideal for a comforting side dish.

11. Coconut Cardamom Rice Pudding:
1. Instructions: Cook rice with coconut milk, cardamom, and a touch of sweetener.
2. Time to Eat: Suitable for a grounding dessert.

12. Spicy Grilled Shrimp Skewers:
1. Instructions: Skewer shrimp with a spicy marinade, grill until cooked through.
2. Time to Eat: Ideal for a comforting dinner.

13. Lemon Mint Quinoa Tabouleh:
1. Instructions: Toss quinoa with fresh mint, lemon juice, and finely chopped veggies.
2. Time to Eat: Suitable for a refreshing lunch.

14. Chai-Spiced Baked Acorn Squash:
1. Instructions: Roast acorn squash with a chai-inspired spice blend until tender.
2. Time to Eat: Ideal for a grounding side dish.

15. Lentil Spinach Curry:
1. Instructions: Cook lentils and spinach with a curry sauce for a hearty meal.
2. Time to Eat: Suitable for a comforting dinner.

16. Ginger Turmeric Grilled Chicken:
1. Instructions: Marinate chicken in a mix of ginger, turmeric, and grill until cooked.
2. Time to Eat: Ideal for a grounding dinner.

17. Rosemary Garlic Roasted Potatoes:
1. Instructions: Roast potatoes with rosemary,

garlic, and a drizzle of olive oil.
2. Time to Eat: Suitable for a comforting side dish.

18. Spiced Berry Chia Pudding:

1. Instructions: Mix chia seeds with a blend of berries and spices for a nourishing pudding.
2. Time to Eat: Ideal for a grounding breakfast or snack.

19. Sesame Ginger Noodle Salad:

1. Instructions: Toss noodles with a sesame-ginger dressing and assorted veggies.
2. Time to Eat: Suitable for a refreshing lunch.

20. Citrus Herb Baked Salmon:

1. Instructions: Bake salmon with a citrus-herb marinade for a flavorful main course.
2. Time to Eat: Ideal for a grounding dinner

21. Cod fillets

1. Instructions: Coat cod fillets in herb seasoning, bake until golden and flaky.
2. Time to Eat: Ideal for a comforting dinner.

22. Quinoa Lentil Stuffed Bell Peppers:

1. Instructions: Fill bell peppers with quinoa, lentils, and a mix of spices, bake until tender.
2. Time to Eat: Suitable for a grounding dinner.

23. Minty Green Pea Soup:

1. Instructions: Blend peas with mint and a hint of lemon for a refreshing soup.
2. Time to Eat: Ideal for a nurturing lunch.

24. Cinnamon Baked Sweet Potato Wedges:

1. Instructions: Roast sweet potato wedges with a dusting of cinnamon until tender.
2. Time to Eat: Suitable for a comforting side

dish.

25. **Ginger Turmeric Carrot Lentil Salad:**
    1. Instructions: Toss cooked lentils, carrots, and ginger-turmeric dressing for a flavorful salad.
    2. Time to Eat: Ideal for a nurturing lunch.

26. **Lemon Thyme Grilled Chicken Skewers:**
    1. Instructions: Skewer chicken with a lemon-thyme marinade, grill until cooked.
    2. Time to Eat: Suitable for a grounding dinner.

27. **Roasted Cauliflower Quinoa Pilaf:**
    1. Instructions: Roast cauliflower, mix with quinoa, and a blend of herbs.
    2. Time to Eat: Ideal for a comforting side dish.

28. **Turmeric Cumin Roasted Veggies:**
    1. Instructions: Roast mixed vegetables with a blend of turmeric and cumin.
    2. Time to Eat: Suitable for a grounding dinner.

29. **Mango Mint Quinoa Salad:**
    1. Instructions: Toss quinoa with fresh mango, mint, and a light vinaigrette.
    2. Time to Eat: Ideal for a refreshing lunch.

30. **Ginger Cardamom Baked Chicken:**
    1. Instructions: Bake chicken with a ginger-cardamom glaze until juicy and aromatic.
    2. Time to Eat: Suitable for a grounding dinner.

31. **Sesame Ginger Glazed Tofu Stir-Fry:**
    1. Instructions: Sauté tofu with a sesame-ginger glaze and colorful veggies.
    2. Time to Eat: Ideal for a comforting dinner.

32. **Spiced Berry Oatmeal:**
    1. Instructions: Mix oats with a medley of

berries and a sprinkle of warming spices.
2. Time to Eat: Suitable for a grounding breakfast.

33. Lemon Turmeric Roasted Brussels Sprouts:
1. Instructions: Roast Brussels sprouts with lemon, turmeric, and a hint of olive oil.
2. Time to Eat: Ideal for a comforting side dish.

34. Tandoori Spiced Roasted Cauliflower:
1. Instructions: Roast cauliflower with a tandoori spice blend for a flavorsome side.
2. Time to Eat: Suitable for a grounding dinner.

35. Lavender Honey Yogurt Parfait:
1. Instructions: Layer yogurt with a drizzle of lavender honey and fresh fruit for a nourishing dessert.
2. Time to Eat: Ideal for a grounding dessert or snack.

36. Saffron Coconut Rice Pilaf:
1. Instructions: Cook rice with saffron and coconut milk for a subtly sweet side.
2. Time to Eat: Suitable for a comforting side dish.

37. Minted Quinoa Lentil Stew:
1. Instructions: Cook quinoa and lentils in a mint-infused broth for a nourishing meal.
2. Time to Eat: Ideal for a comforting lunch.

38. Cardamom Honey Roasted Carrots:
1. Instructions: Roast carrots with a cardamom-infused honey glaze.
2. Time to Eat: Suitable for a grounding side dish.

39. Chai-Spiced Baked Pears:
1. Instructions: Bake pears with a chai-inspired

spice blend until tender and fragrant.

2. Time to Eat: Ideal for a comforting dessert.

40. **Saffron-infused Vegetable Paella:** and fragrant.

1. Instructions: Cook a medley of vegetables and saffron-infused rice for a vibrant meal.
2. Time to Eat: Suitable for a grounding dinner.

These recipes offer a diverse mix of flavors and ingredients designed to balance all three doshas. Adjust serving sizes and ingredients based on individual tastes and dietary needs.

In the pages of "Dosha Dining: 300 Recipes for Balanced Wellness," the journey through the world of Ayurvedic culinary wisdom culminates in a celebration of harmony, nourishment, and well-being. Each recipe has been thoughtfully crafted to align with the unique needs of Vata, Pitta, and Kapha doshas, unlocking a tapestry of flavors that not only delight the palate but also restore equilibrium within.

As we conclude this flavorful odyssey, may these recipes continue to serve as a compass, guiding us toward balance and vitality. Let this collection stand as a culinary companion, always ready to aid us in embracing a lifestyle where every meal is an opportunity for rejuvenation, balance, and holistic wellness. Here's to savoring the flavors of well-being and crafting a nourishing harmony in our everyday lives.